Dash Diet Cookbook for Busy people

50 Affordable and Inspired Meals to Stay Fit and Healthy with Taste

Natalie Puckett

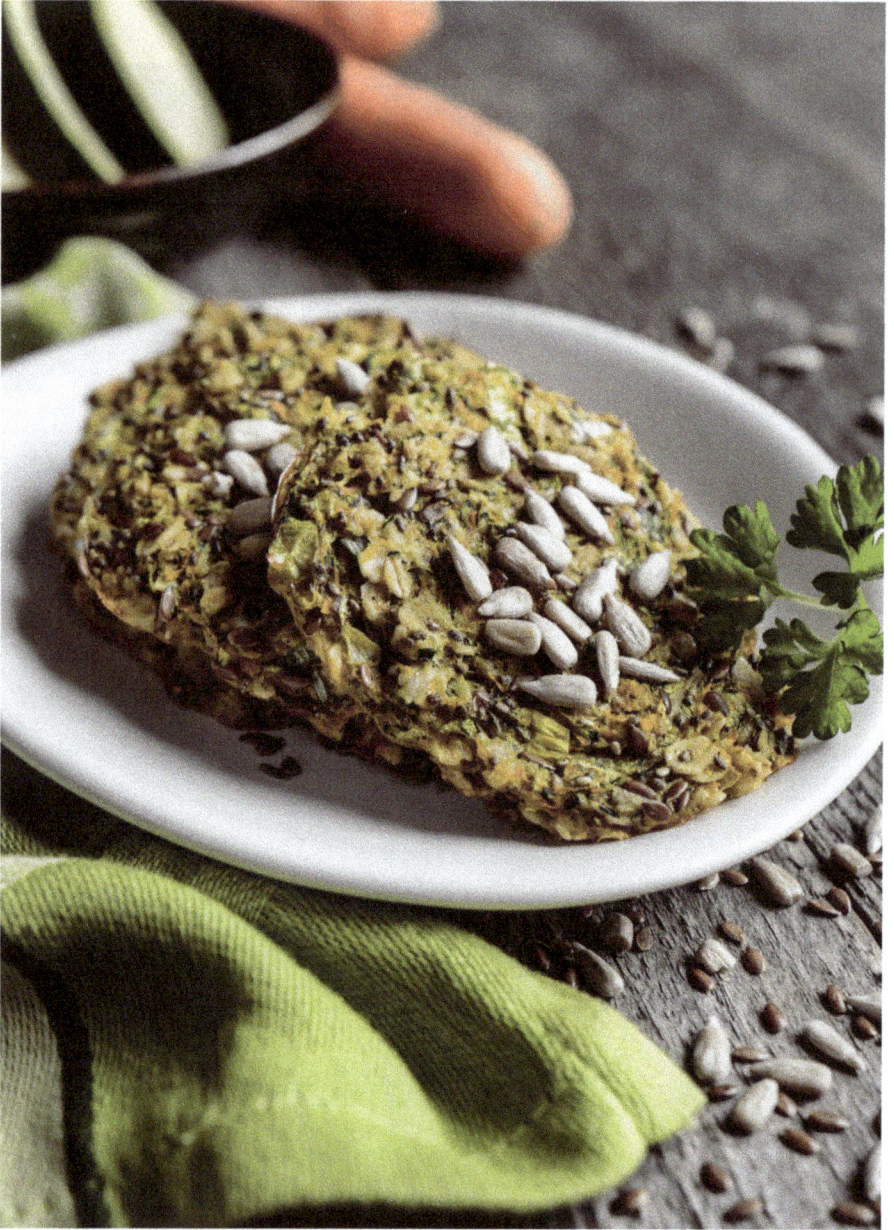

Table of Contents

Carrot and Zucchini Oatmeal

Serving: 3

Prep Time: 10 minutes

Cook Time: 8 hours

Ingredients:

½ cup steel cut oats

1 cup coconut milk

1 carrot, grated

¼ zucchini, grated

Pinch of nutmeg

½ teaspoon cinnamon powder

2 tablespoons brown sugar

¼ cup pecans, chopped

How To:

1.   Grease the Slow Cooker well.

2.   Add oats, zucchini, milk, carrot, nutmeg, cloves, sugar, cinnamon and stir well.

3. Place lid and cook on LOW for 8 hours.

4. Divide amongst serving bowls and enjoy!

Nutrition (Per Serving)

Calories: 200

Fat: 4g

Carbohydrates: 11g

Protein: 5g

Blueberry and Walnut "Steel" Oatmeal

Serving: 8

Prep Time: 5 minutes

Cook Time: 7-8 hours

Ingredients:

2 cups steel-cut oats

6 cups water

2 cups low-fat milk

2 cups fresh blueberries

1 ripe banana, mashed

1 teaspoon vanilla extract

2 teaspoons ground cinnamon

2 tablespoons brown sugar

Pinch of salt

½ cup walnuts, chopped

How To:

1.   Grease the within of your Slow Cooker.

2.   Add oats, milk, water, blueberries, banana, vanilla, sugar, cinnamon and salt to your Slow Cooker.

3.   Stir.

4.   Place lid and cook on LOW for 7-8 hours.

5.   Serve warm with a garnish of chopped walnuts.

6.   Enjoy!

Nutrition (Per Serving)

Calories: 372

Fat: 14g

Carbohydrates: 56g

Protein: 8g

Shrimp and Egg Medley

Serving: 4

Prep Time: 15 minutes

Cook Time: nil

Ingredients:

4 hardboiled eggs, peeled and chopped

1-pound cooked shrimp, peeled and de-veined, chopped

1 sprig fresh dill, chopped

¼ cup mayonnaise

1 teaspoon Dijon mustard

4 fresh lettuce leaves

How To:

1.   Take an outsized serving bowl and add the listed ingredients (except lettuce.)

2.   Stir well.

3.   Serve over bet of lettuce leaves.

4.   Enjoy!

Nutrition (Per Serving)

Calories: 292

Fat: 17g

Carbohydrates: 1.6g

Protein: 30g

Crispy Walnut Crumbles

Serving: 10

Prep Time: 10 minutes

Cook Time: 8 minutes

Ingredients:

6 ounces kite ricotta/cashew cheese, grated

2 tablespoons walnuts, chopped

1 tablespoon almond butter

½ tablespoon fresh thyme chopped

How To:

1.   Preheat your oven to 350 degrees F.

2.   Take two large rimmed baking sheets and line with parchment.

3.   Add cheese, almond butter to a kitchen appliance and blend.

4.   Add walnuts to the combination and pulse.

5.   Take a tablespoon and scoop mix onto a baking sheet.

6.   Top them with chopped thymes.

7.   Bake for 8 minutes, transfer to a cooling rack.

8.   Let it cool for half-hour.

9.   Serve and enjoy!

Nutrition (Per Serving)

Calories: 80

Fat: 3g

Carbohydrates: 7g

Protein: 7g

Cheesy Zucchini Omelette

Serving: 3

Prep Time: 10 minutes

Cook Time: 20 minutes

Ingredients:

4 large eggs

2-3 medium zucchinis

1-2 garlic cloves, crushed

4 tablespoons grated cheese Season as needed

How To:

1.   Take a bowl and add grated zucchinis, confirm to peel them because the skin is bitter.

2.   Take a bowl and break within the eggs, crushed garlic and cheese.

3.   Pour the mixture during a hot frypan with a touch little bit of oil and place it over medium heat, keep a lid on.

4.   Once the egg is cooked nicely, and therefore the bottom is crispy and golden, serve and luxuriate in with a garnish of chopped parsley.

5.   Enjoy!

Nutrition (Per Serving)

Calories: 289

Fat: 20g

Carbohydrates: 7g

Protein: 21g

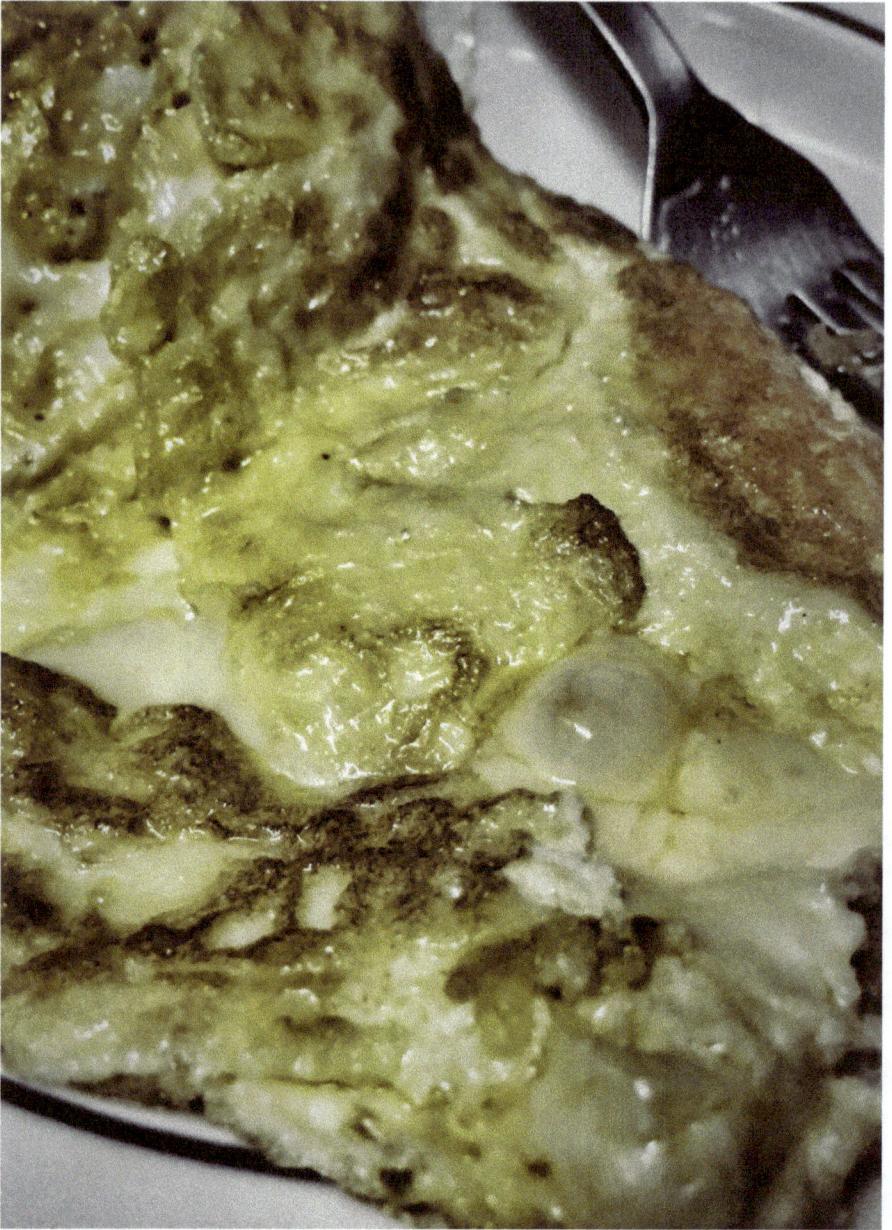

Old Fashioned Breakfast Oatmeal

Serving: 4

Prep Time: 10 minutes

Cook Time: 5 minutes

Ingredients:

2 ½ cups water

1 cup old fashioned oats

1 cup apple, peeled, cored and chopped

3 tablespoons low-fat butter

2 tablespoons palm sugar

½ teaspoon cinnamon powder

How To:

1. Add water, oats, apple, butter, cinnamon, and sugar to a moment pot.

2. Toss well and lock the lid.

3. Cook on high for five minutes.

4. Release the pressure naturally over 10 minutes.

5.   Stir oats and divide into bowls.

6.   Enjoy!

Nutrition (Per Serving)

Calories: 191

Fat: 2g

Carbohydrates: 9g

Protein: 5g

Healthy Peach Oatmeal

Serving: 8

Prep Time: 10 minutes

Cook Time: 10 minutes

Ingredients:

4 cups old fashioned rolled oats

3 ½ cups low-fat milk

3 ½ cups water

1 teaspoon cinnamon powder

1/3 cup palm sugar

4 peaches, chopped

How To:

1.　　Add oats, milk, cinnamon, water, sugar, and peaches to your Instant Pot.

2.　　Toss well.

3.　　Lock the lid and cook for 10 minutes on high.

4.　　Release the pressure naturally over 10 minutes.

5.   Divide the combination in bowls and serve!

Nutrition (Per Serving)

Calories: 192

Fat: 3g

Carbohydrates: 12g

Protein: 4g

Crazy Lamb Salad

Serving: 4

Prep Time: 10 minutes

Cook Time: 35 minutes

Ingredients:

1 tablespoon olive oil

3-pound leg of lamb, bone removed, leg butterflied Salt and pepper to taste

1 teaspoon cumin

Pinch of dried thyme

2 garlic cloves, peeled and minced For Salad

4 ounces feta cheese, crumbled

½ cup pecans

2 cups spinach

1 ½ tablespoons lemon juice

¼ cup olive oil

1 cup fresh mint, chopped

How To:

1.   Rub lamb with salt and pepper, 1 tablespoon oil, thyme, cumin, minced garlic.

2.   Pre-heat your grill to medium-high and transfer lamb.

3.   Cook for 40 minutes, ensuring to flip it once.

4.   Take a lined baking sheet and spread the pecans.

5.   Toast in oven for 10 minutes at 350 degree F.

6.   Transfer grilled lamb to chopping board and let it cool.

7.   Slice.

8.   Take a salad bowl and add spinach, 1 cup mint, feta cheese, ¼ cup vegetable oil , juice , toasted pecans, salt, pepper and toss well.

9.   Add lamb slices on top.

10.   Serve and enjoy!

Nutrition (Per Serving)

Calories: 334

Fat: 33g

Carbohydrates: 5g

Protein: 7g

Hearty Roasted Cauliflower

Serving: 8

Prep Time: 5 minutes

Cook Time: 30 minutes

Ingredients:

1 large cauliflower head

2 tablespoons melted coconut oil

2 tablespoons fresh thyme

1 teaspoon Celtic sea sunflower seeds

1 teaspoon fresh ground pepper

1 head roasted garlic

2 tablespoons fresh thyme for garnish

How To:

1.   Pre-heat your oven to 425 degrees F.

2.   Rinse cauliflower and trim, core and sliced.

3.   Lay cauliflower evenly on rimmed baking tray.

4.   Drizzle copra oil evenly over cauliflower, sprinkle thyme leaves.

5.   Season with pinch of sunflower seeds and pepper.

6.   Squeeze roasted garlic.

7.   Roast cauliflower until slightly caramelized for about half-hour, ensuring to show once.

8.   Garnish with fresh thyme leaves.

9.   Enjoy!

Nutrition (Per Serving)

Calories: 129

Fat: 11g

Carbohydrates: 6g

Protein: 7g

Cool Cabbage Fried Beef

Serving: 4

Prep Time: 5 minutes

Cook Time: 15 minutes

Ingredients:

1-pound beef, ground and lean

½ pound bacon

1 onion

1 garlic clove, minced

½ head cabbage

pepper to taste

How To:

1.   Take skillet and place it over medium heat.

2.   Add chopped bacon, beef and onion until slightly browned.

3.   Transfer to a bowl and keep it covered.

4.   Add minced garlic and cabbage to the skillet and cook

until slightly browned.

5. Return the bottom beef mix to the skillet and simmer for 3-5 minutes over low heat.

6. Serve and enjoy!

Nutrition (Per Serving)

Calories: 360

Fat: 22g

Net Carbohydrates: 5g

Protein: 34g

Fennel and Figs Lamb

Serving: 2

Prep Time: 10 minutes

Cook Time: 40 minutes

Ingredients:

6 ounces lamb racks 1 fennel bulbs, sliced pepper to taste

1 tablespoon olive oil

2 figs, cut in half

1/8 cup apple cider vinegar

1/2 tablespoon swerve

How To:

1.   Take a bowl and add fennel, figs, vinegar, swerve, oil and toss.

2.   Transfer to baking dish.

3.   Season with sunflower seeds and pepper.

4.   Bake for quarter-hour at 400 degrees F.

5.   Season lamb with sunflower seeds and pepper and transfer to a heated pan over medium-high heat.

6.   Cook for a couple of minutes.

7.   Add lamb to the baking dish with fennel and bake for 20 minutes.

8.   Divide between plates and serve.

9.   Enjoy!

Nutrition (Per Serving)

Calories: 230

Fat: 3g

Carbohydrates: 5g

Protein: 10g

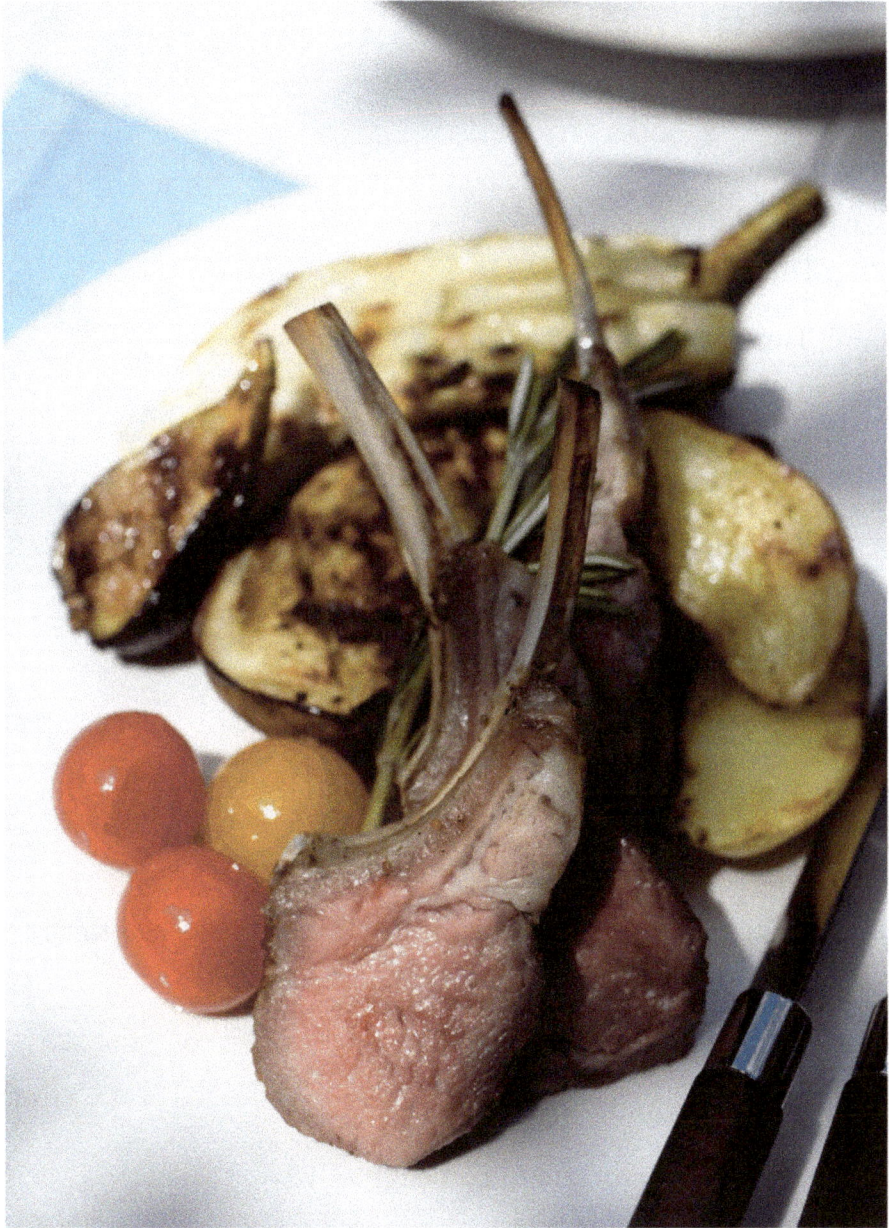

Black Berry Chicken Wings

Serving: 4

Prep Time: 35 minutes

Cook Time: 50minutes

Ingredients:

3 pounds chicken wings, about 20 pieces ½ cup blackberry chipotle jam Pepper to taste

½ cup water

How To:

1.   Add water and jam to a bowl and blend well.

2.   Place chicken wings during a zip bag and add two-thirds of marinade.

3.   Season with pepper.

4.   Let it marinate for half-hour.

5.   Pre-heat your oven to 400 degrees F.

6.   Prepare a baking sheet and wire rack, place chicken wings in wire rack and bake for quarter-hour.

7.   Brush remaining marinade and bake for half-hour more.

8.   Enjoy!

Nutrition (Per Serving)

Calories: 502

Fat: 39g

Carbohydrates: 01.8g

Protein: 34g

Mushroom and Olive "Mediterranean" Steak

Serving: 2

Prep Time: 10 minutes

Cook Time: 14 minutes

Ingredients:

1/2-pound boneless beef sirloin steak, ¾ inch thick, cut into 4 pieces

1/2 large red onion, chopped

1/2 cup mushrooms

2 garlic cloves, thinly sliced

2 tablespoons olive oil

1/4 cup green olives, coarsely chopped

1/2 cup parsley leaves, finely cut

How To:

Take an outsized sized skillet and place it over medium-high heat.

1. Add oil and let it heat up.

2. Add beef and cook until each side are browned, remove beef and drain fat.

3. Add the remainder of the oil to the skillet and warmth.

4. Add onions, garlic and cook for 2-3 minutes.

5. Stir well.

6. Add mushrooms, olives and cook until the mushrooms are thoroughly done.

7. Return the meat to the skillet and reduce heat to medium.

8. Cook for 3-4 minutes (covered).

9. Stir in parsley.

10. Serve and enjoy!

Nutrition (Per Serving)

Calories: 386

Fat: 30g

Carbohydrates: 11g

Protein: 21g

Orange and Chili Garlic Sauce

Serving: 5 cups

Prep Time: 15 minutes

Cook Time: 8 hours

Ingredients:

½ cup apple cider vinegar

4 pounds red jalapeno peppers, stems, seeds and ribs removed, chopped

10 garlic cloves, chopped

½ cup tomato paste

Juice of 1 orange zest

½ cup honey

2 tablespoons soy sauce

2 teaspoons salt

How To:

1.   Add vinegar, garlic, peppers, ingredient , fruit juice , honey, zest, soy and salt to your Slow Cooker.

2.   Stir and shut lid.

3.   Cook on LOW for 8 hours.

4.   Use as required!

Nutrition (Per Serving)

Calories: 33

Fat: 1g

Carbohydrates: 8g

Protein: 1g

Tantalizing Mushroom Gravy

Serving: 2 cups

Prep Time: 5 minutes

Cook Time: 5-8 hours

Ingredients:

1 cup button mushrooms, sliced

¾ cup low-fat buttermilk

1/3 cup water

1 medium onion, finely diced

2 garlic cloves, minced

2 tablespoons extra virgin olive oil

2 tablespoons all-purpose flour

1 tablespoon fresh rosemary, minced Freshly ground black pepper

How To:

1.   Add the listed ingredients to your Slow Cooker.

2.   Place lid and cook on LOW for 5-8 hours.

3.   Serve warm and use as needed!

Nutrition (Per Serving)

Calories: 54

Fat: 4g

Carbohydrates: 4g

Protein: 2g

Everyday Vegetable Stock

Serving: 10 cups

Prep Time: 5 minutes

Cook Time: 8-12 hours

Ingredients:

2 celery stalks (with leaves), quartered

4 ounces mushrooms, with stems

2 carrots, unpeeled and quartered

1 onion, unpeeled, quartered from pole to pole

1 garlic head, unpeeled, halved across middle

2 fresh thyme sprigs

10 peppercorns

½ teaspoon salt

Enough water to fill 3 quarters of Slow Cooker

How To:

1.   Add celery, mushrooms, onion, carrots, garlic, thyme, salt, peppercorn and water to your Slow Cooker.

2.   Stir and canopy.

3.   Cook on LOW for 8-12 hours.

4.   Strain the stock through a fine mesh cloth/metal mesh and discard solids.

5.   Use as needed.

Nutrition (Per Serving)

Calories: 38

Fat: 5g

Carbohydrates: 1g

Protein: 0g

Grilled Chicken with Lemon and Fennel

Serving: 4

Prep Time: 5 minutes

Cook Time: 25 minutes

Ingredients:

2 cups chicken fillets, cut and skewed

1 large fennel bulb

2 garlic cloves

1 jar green olives

1 lemon

How To:

1.   Pre-heat your grill to medium-high.

2.   Crush garlic cloves.

3.   Take a bowl and add vegetable oil and season with sunflower seeds and pepper.

4.   Coat chicken skewers with the marinade.

5.   Transfer them under the grill and grill for 20 minutes, ensuring to show them halfway through until golden.

6.   Zest half the lemon and cut the opposite half into quarters.

7.   Cut the fennel bulb into similarly sized segments.

8.   Brush vegetable oil everywhere the clove segments and cook for 3-5 minutes.

9.   Chop them and add them to the bowl with the marinade.

10.   Add lemon peel and olives.

11.   Once the meat is prepared, serve with the

vegetable mix.

12.   Enjoy!

Nutrition (Per Serving)

Calories: 649

Fat: 16g

Carbohydrates: 33g

Protein: 18g

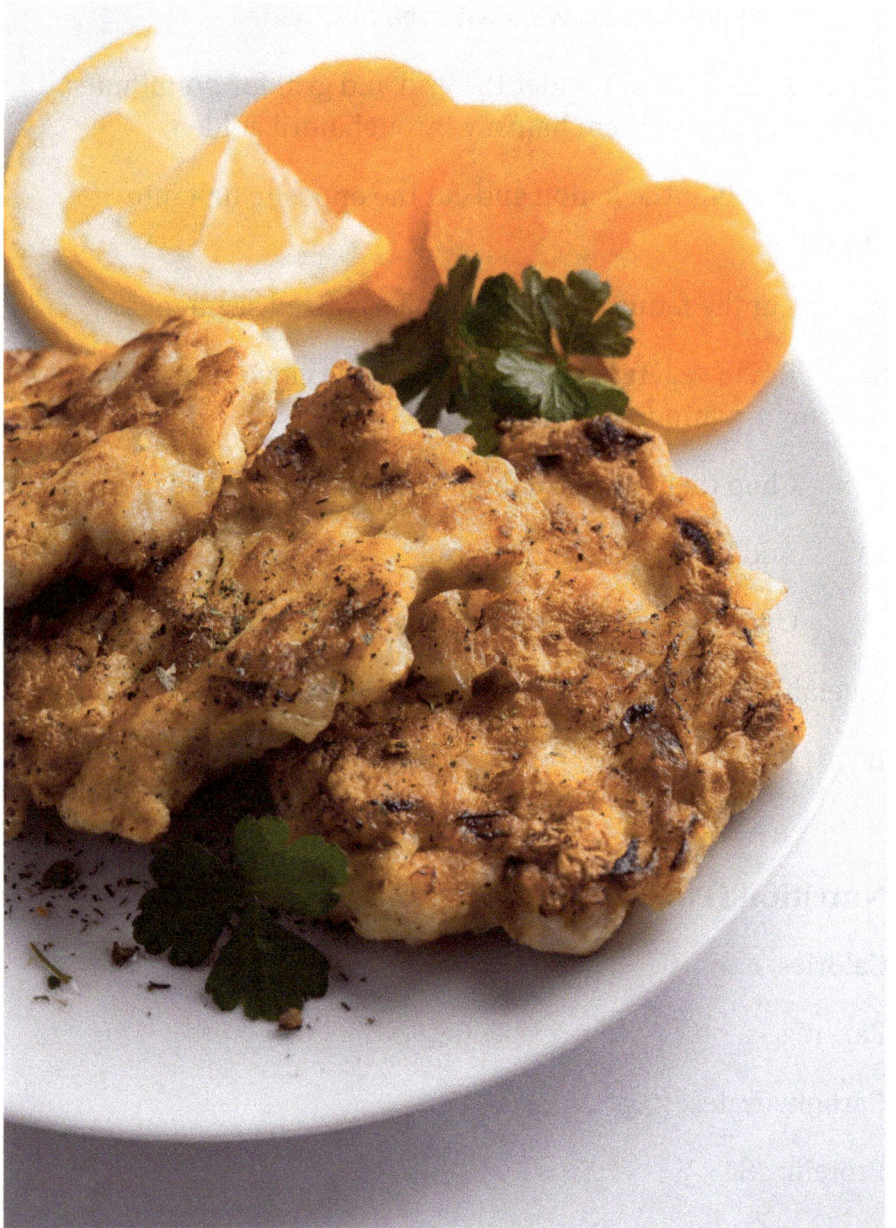

Caramelized Pork Chops and Onion

Serving: 4

Prep Time: 5 minutes

Cook Time: 40 minutes

Ingredients:

4-pound chuck roast

4 ounces green Chili, chopped

2 tablespoons of chili powder

½ teaspoon of dried oregano

½ teaspoon of cumin, ground

2 garlic cloves, minced

How To:

1.   Rub the chops with a seasoning of 1 teaspoon of pepper and a couple of teaspoons of sunflower seeds.

2.   Take a skillet and place it over medium heat, add oil and

permit the oil to heat up.

3.   Brown the seasoned chop each side.

4.   Add water and onion to the skillet and canopy , lower the warmth to low and simmer for 20 minutes.

5.   Turn the chops over and season with more sunflower seeds and pepper.

6.   Cover and cook until the water fully evaporates and therefore the beer [MOU1] shows a rather brown texture.

7.   Remove the chops and serve with a topping of the caramelized onion.

8.   Serve and enjoy!

Nutrition (Per Serving)

Calorie: 47

Fat: 4g

Carbohydrates: 4g

Protein: 0.5g

Healthy Cauliflower Salad

Serving: 4

Prep Time: 10 minutes

Cook Time: nil

Ingredients:

1 head cauliflower, broken into florets

1 small onion, chopped

1/8 cup extra virgin olive oil

¼ cup apple cider vinegar

½ teaspoon sea salt

½ teaspoon black pepper

¼ cup dried cranberries

¼ cup pumpkin seeds

How To:

1.   Wash the cauliflower thoroughly and break down into florets.

2.   Transfer the florets to a bowl.

3.   Take another bowl and whisk in oil, salt, pepper and vinegar.

4.   Add pumpkin seeds, cranberries to the bowl with dressing.

5.   Mix well and pour dressing over cauliflower florets.

6.   Toss well.

7.   Add onions and toss.

8.   Chill and serve.

9.   Enjoy!

Nutrition (Per Serving)

Calories: 163

Fat: 11g

Carbohydrates: 16g

Protein: 3g

Chickpea Salad

Serving: 4

Prep Time: 6 minutes

Cook Time: Nil

Ingredients:

1 cup canned chickpeas, drained and rinsed.

2 spring onions, thinly sliced.

1 small cucumber, diced.

2 green bell peppers, chopped.

2 tomatoes, diced.

2 tablespoons fresh parsley, chopped.

1 teaspoon capers, drained and rinsed.

Half a lemon, juiced.

2 tablespoons sunflower oil.

1 tablespoon red wine vinegar.

Pinch of dried oregano.

Sunflower seeds and pepper to taste

How To:

1.   Take a medium sized bowl and add chickpeas, spring onions, cucumber, bell pepper, tomato, parsley and capers.

2.   Take another bowl and mix in the rest of the ingredients, pour mixture over chickpea salad and toss well.

3.   Coat and serve, enjoy!

Nutrition (Per Serving)

Calories: 74

Fat: 0.7g

Carbohydrates: 16g

Protein: 2g

Dashing Bok Choy Samba

Serving: 3

Prep Time: 5 minutes

Cook Time: 15 minutes

Ingredients:

4 bok choy, sliced

1 onion, sliced

½ cup Parmesan cheese, grated

4 teaspoons coconut cream

Sunflower seeds and freshly ground black pepper, to taste

How To:

1.   Mix bok choy with black pepper and sunflower seeds.

2.   Take a cooking pan, heat the oil and to sauté sliced onion for 5 minutes.

3.   Then add cream and seasoned bok choy.

4.   Cook for 6 minutes.

5.   Stir in Parmesan cheese and cover with a lid.

6.   Reduce the heat to low and cook for 3 minutes.

7.   Serve warm and enjoy!

Nutrition (Per Serving)

Calories: 112

Fat: 4.9g

Carbohydrates: 1.9g

Protein: 3g

Simple Avocado Caprese Salad

Serving: 6

Prep Time: 15 minutes

Cook Time: 29 minutes

Ingredients:

2 avocados, cubed

1 cup cherry tomatoes, halved

8 ounces mozzarella balls, halved

2 tablespoons finely chopped fresh basil

2 tablespoons olive oil

2 tablespoons balsamic vinegar

1 tablespoon sunflower seeds Fresh ground black pepper

How To:

1. Take a bowl and add the listed ingredients, toss them well until thoroughly mixed.

2.   Season with pepper according to your taste.

3.   Serve and enjoy!

Nutrition (Per Serving)

Calories: 358

Fat: 30g

Carbohydrates: 9g

Protein: 14g

The Rutabaga Wedge Dish

Serving: 4

Prep Time: 15 minutes

Cook Time: 45 minutes

Ingredients:

2 medium rutabagas, medium, cleaned and peeled

4 tablespoons almond butter

½ teaspoon sunflower seeds

½ teaspoon onion powder

1/8 teaspoon black pepper

½ cup buffalo wing sauce

¼ cup blue cheese dressing, low fat and low sodium 2 green onions, chopped

How To:

1.   Pre-heat your oven to 400 degrees F.

2.   Line a baking sheet with parchment paper.

3. Wash and peel rutabagas, clean and peel them, and cut into wedge shapes.

4. Take a skillet and place it over low heat, add almond butter and melt.

5. Stir in onion powder, sunflower seeds, onion, black pepper.

6. Use seasoned almond butter to coat wedges.

7. Arrange wedges in a single layer on the baking sheet.

8. Bake for 30 minutes.

9. Remove and coat in buffalo sauce and return to oven.

10. Bake for 15 minutes more.

11. Place wedges on serving plate and trickle with blue cheese dressing.

12. Garnish with chopped green onion and enjoy!

Nutrition (Per Serving)

Calories: 235

Fat: 15g

Carbohydrates: 10g

Protein: 2.5g

Red Coleslaw

Serving: 4

Prep Time: 10 minutes

Cook Time: 0 minutes

Ingredients:

1 2/3 pounds red cabbage

2 tablespoons ground caraway seeds

1 tablespoon whole grain mustard

1 1/4 cups mayonnaise

Sunflower seeds and black pepper

How To:

1. Take a large bowl and all the remaining ingredients.

2. Mix it well and let it sit for 10 minutes.

3. Serve and enjoy!

Nutrition (Per Serving)

Calories: 406

Fat: 40.8g

Carbohydrates: 10g

Protein: 2.2g

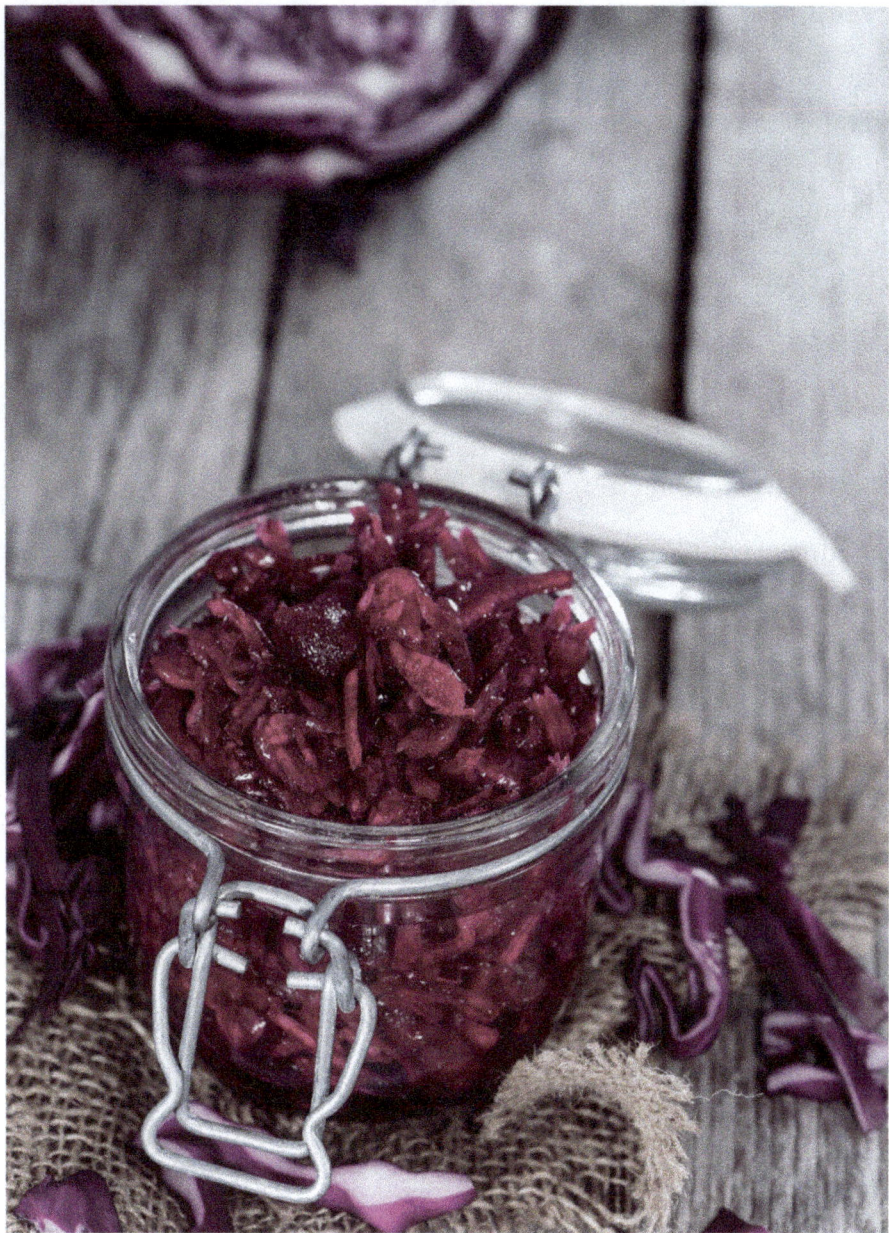

Classic Tuna Salad

Serving: 4

Prep Time: 10 minutes

Cook Time: Nil

Ingredients:

12 ounces white tuna, in water

½ cup celery, diced

2 tablespoons fresh parsley, chopped

2 tablespoons low-calorie mayonnaise, low fat and low sodium

½ teaspoon Dijon mustard

½ teaspoon sunflower seeds

¼ teaspoon fresh ground black pepper

Direction

1.   Take a medium sized bowl and add tuna, parsley, and celery.

2.   Mix well and add mayonnaise and mustard.

3.   Season with pepper and sunflower seeds.

4.   Stir and add olives, relish, chopped pickle, onion and mix well.

5.   Serve and enjoy

Nutrition (Per Serving)

Calories: 137

Fat: 5g

Carbohydrates: 1g

Protein: 20g

Panko-Crusted Cod

Prep time: 10 minutes

Cook time: 15 minutes

Servings: 2

Ingredients

Panko-style breadcrumbs – ¼ cup Garlic - 1 clove, minced
Extra-virgin olive oil – 1 Tbsp. Nonfat Greek yogurt – 3 Tbsp.
Mayonnaise – 1 Tbsp.

Lemon juice – 1 ½ tsp.

Tarragon – ½ tsp.

Pinch of salt

Cod – 10 ounces, cut into two portions

Method

1.   Preheat the oven to 425F.

2.   Coat a baking pan with cooking spray.

3.   In a bowl, combine olive oil, garlic, and breadcrumbs.

4.   In another bowl, combine lemon juice, mayonnaise,
yogurt, tarragon, and salt.

5.   Place fish in the baking pan. Top each piece with one-half yogurt mixture then 1/3 breadcrumb mixture.

6.   Bake in the oven for 15 minutes.

7.   Serve.

Nutritional Facts Per Serving

Calories: 225

Fat: 10g

Carb: 13g

Protein: 18g

Sodium 270mg

Grilled Salmon and Asparagus with Lemon Butter

Prep time: 10 minutes

Cook time: 20 minutes

Servings: 4

Ingredients

Salmon – 1 ¼ pound, cut into 4 portions Asparagus – 2 bunches, ends trimmed Olive oil cooking spray Salt – ½ tsp. Freshly ground black pepper – ¼ tsp. Garlic powder – ¼ tsp. Olive oil – 1 Tbsp.

Butter – 1 Tbsp.

Lemon juice – 3 Tbsp.

Method

1.   On a baking sheet, place the salmon and asparagus. Spray lightly with cooking spray. Season with salt, pepper, and garlic powder.

2.   Grease and preheat grill. Place salmon and asparagus on it.

3.   Grill total 6 minutes, 3 minutes per side, or until opaque, turning once.

4.   Grill the asparagus for 5 to 7 minutes, or until tender, turning occasionally.

5.   In a bowl, place butter, olive oil, and lemon juice. Microwave to melt.

6.   Drizzle fish with this mixture.

7.   Serve.

Nutritional Facts Per Serving

Calories: 190

Fat: 8g

Carb: 6g

Protein: 24g

Sodium 445mg

Pan-Roasted Fish Fillets with Herb Butter

Prep time: 10 minutes

Cook time: 5 minutes

Servings: 2

Ingredients

Fish fillets – 2 (5-ounce each) ½ to 1-inch-thick Salt – ¼ tsp.

Ground black pepper Olive oil – 3 Tbsp.

Unsalted butter -1 Tbsp. divided

Fresh thyme – 2 sprigs

Chopped flat-leaf parsley - 1 Tbsp. Lemon wedges

Method

1.   Rub the fish with pepper and salt.

2.   Heat oil in a skillet.

3.   Place fillets and cook until around the edges, about 2 to 3 minutes. Then flip the fillets and add the butter and thyme to the pan.

4.   Baste the fish with melted butter until golden all over, about 2 minutes.

5.   Serve with chopped parsley and lemon wedges.

Nutritional Facts Per Serving

Calories: 369

Fat: 26.9g

Carb: 1g

Protein: 30.5g

Sodium 62mg

Chili Macadamia Crusted Tilapia

Prep time: 20 minutes

Cook time: 7 minutes

Servings: 4

Ingredients

Tilapia fillets – 4

Macadamia nuts – ½ cup, chopped coarsely

Whole wheat panko crumbs – ½ cup Chili powder – 1 tsp.

Cayenne pepper – ¼ tsp.

Paprika – ¼ tsp.

Salt – ¼ tsp.

Pepper – ¼ tsp.

Egg – 1

Olive oil – 3 Tbsp.

Method

1. In a bowl, combine panko crumbs, nuts, chili powder, cayenne pepper, paprika, salt, and pepper.

2. Whisk egg in another bowl and set aside.

3. Heat the olive oil in a skillet.

4. Dredge each tilapia fillet in the egg and then coat it in the macadamia-spice-panko mixture.

5. Cook fillets until browned and cooked through, about 3 minutes on each side.

6. Serve.

Nutritional Facts Per Serving

Calories: 351

Fat: 26.5g

Carb: 5.7g

Protein: 25.7g

Sodium 234mg

Broiled White Sea Bass

Prep time: 5 minutes

Cook time: 10 minutes

Servings: 2

Ingredients

White sea bass fillets – 2, each 4 ounces Lemon juice – 1 Tbsp. Garlic – 1 tsp. minced

Salt-free herb seasoning blend – ¼ tsp. Ground black pepper to taste

Method

1.   Heat the broiler (grill).

2.   Place the rack very close (4 inches) to the heat source.

3.   Place the fillets in a greased baking pan.

4.   Sprinkle the fillets with herbed seasoning, garlic, lemon juice, and pepper.

5.   Broil (grill) until opaque throughout, about 8 to 10 minutes

6.   Serve.

Nutritional Facts Per Serving

Calories: 102

Fat: 2g

Carb: 1g

Protein: 21g

Sodium 77mg

Grilled Asian Salmon

Prep time: 1 hour

Cook time: 10 minutes

Servings: 4

Ingredients

Sesame oil – 1 Tbsp.

Homemade soy sauce – 1 Tbsp.

Fresh ginger – 1 Tbsp. minced Rice wine vinegar – 1 Tbsp.

Salmon fillets – 4, each 4 ounces

Method

1.   Combine vinegar, ginger, soy sauce, and sesame oil in a dish.

2.   Add salmon and coat well. Marinate for 1 hour, turning occasionally (in the refrigerator).

3.   Grease a grill and heat over medium heat.

4.   Grill the salmon on 5 minutes per side or until almost opaque.

5.   Serve.

Nutritional Facts Per Serving

Calories: 185

Fat: 9g

Carb: 1g

Protein: 26g

Sodium 113mg

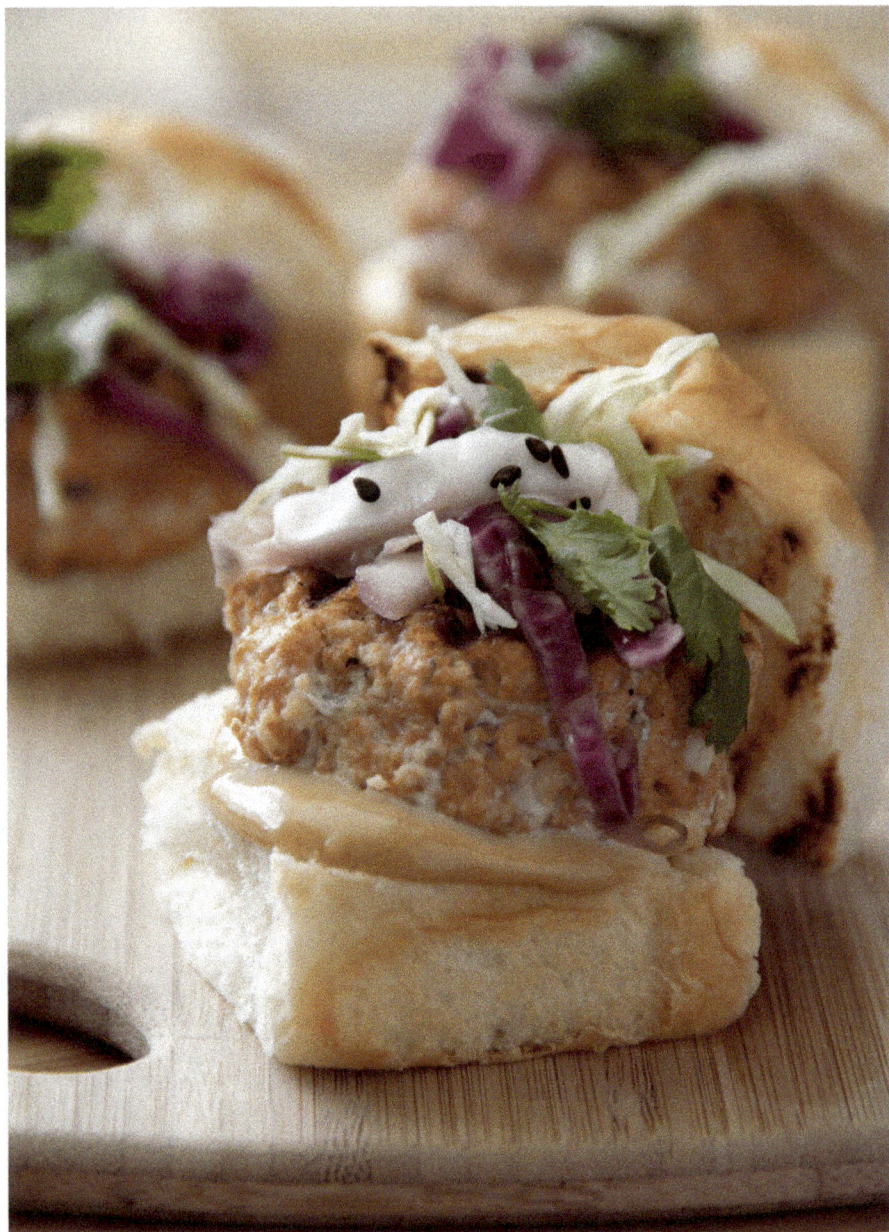

Pumpkin Pie Fat Bombs

Serving: 12

Prep Time: 35 minutes

Cooking Time: 5 minutes

Freeze Time: 3 hours

Ingredients:

2 tablespoons coconut oil

1/3 cup pumpkin puree

1/3 cup almond oil

¼ cup almond oil

3 ounces sugar-free dark chocolate

1 ½ teaspoons pumpkin pie spice mix Stevia to taste

How To:

1.	Melt almond oil and dark chocolate over a double boiler.

2.	Take this mixture and layer the bottom of 12 muffin cups.

3.	Freeze until the crust has set.

4.   Meanwhile, take a saucepan and combine the rest of the ingredients.

5.   Put the saucepan on low heat.

6.   Heat until softened and mix well.

7.   Pour this over the initial chocolate mixture.

8.   Let it chill for at least 1 hour.

Nutrition (Per Serving)

Total Carbs: 3g

Fiber: 1g

Protein: 3g

Fat: 13g

Calories: 124

Sensational Lemonade Fat Bomb

Serving: 2

Prep Time: 2 hours

Cook Time: Nil

Ingredients:

½ lemon

4 ounces cream cheese

2 ounces almond butter

Salt to taste

2 teaspoons natural sweetener

How To:

1.   Take a fine grater and zest lemon.

2.   Squeeze lemon juice into bowl with zest.

3.   Add butter, cream cheese in a bowl and add zest, juice, salt, sweetener.

4.   Mix well using a hand mixer until smooth.

5.   Spoon mixture into molds and let them freeze for 2 hours.

6.   Serve and enjoy!

Nutrition (Per Serving)

Calories: 404

Fat: 43g

Carbohydrates: 4g

Protein: 4g

Sweet Almond and Coconut Fat Bombs

Serving: 6

Prep Time: 10 minutes

Cooking Time: / Freeze Time: 20 minutes

Ingredients:

¼ cup melted coconut oil

9 ½ tablespoons almond butter

90 drops liquid stevia

3 tablespoons cocoa

9 tablespoons melted butter, salted

How To:

1.   Take a bowl and add all of the listed ingredients.

2.   Mix them well.

3.   Pour scant 2 tablespoons of the mixture into as many muffin molds as you like.

4.   Chill for 20 minutes and pop them out.

5.   Serve and enjoy!

Nutrition (Per Serving)

Total Carbs: 2g

Fiber: 0g

Protein: 2.53g

Fat: 14g

Almond and Tomato Balls

Serving: 6

Prep Time: 10 minutes

Cooking Time: / Freeze Time: 20 minutes

Ingredients:

1/3 cup pistachios, de-shelled

10 ounces cream cheese

1/3 cup sun dried tomatoes, diced

How To:

1.   Chop pistachios into small pieces.

2.   Add cream cheese, tomatoes in a bowl and mix well.

3.   Chill for 15-20 minutes and turn into balls.

4.   Roll into pistachios.

5.   Serve and enjoy!

Nutrition (Per Serving)

Carb: 183

Fat: 18g

Carb: 5g

Protein: 5g

Avocado Tuna Bites

Serving: 4

Prep Time: 10 minutes

Cook Time: nil

Ingredients:

1/3 cup coconut oil

1 avocado, cut into cubes

10 ounces canned tuna, drained

¼ cup parmesan cheese, grated

¼ teaspoon garlic powder

1/4 teaspoon onion powder

1/3 cup almond flour

¼ teaspoon pepper

¼ cup low fat mayonnaise Pepper as needed

How To:

1.   Take a bowl and add tuna, mayo, flour, parmesan, spices and mix well.

2.   Fold in avocado and make 12 balls out of the mixture.

3.   Melt coconut oil in pan and cook over medium heat, until all sides are golden.

4.   Serve and enjoy!

Nutrition (Per Serving)

Calories: 185

Fat: 18g

Carbohydrates: 1g

Protein: 5g

Mediterranean Pop Corn Bites

Serving: 4

Prep Time: 5 minutes + 20 minutes chill time

Cook Time: 2-3 minutes

Ingredients:

3 cups Medjool dates, chopped

12 ounces brewed coffee 1 cup pecan, chopped ½ cup coconut, shredded ½ cup cocoa powder

How To:

1.   Soak dates in warm coffee for 5 minutes.

2.   Remove dates from coffee and mash them, making a fine smooth mixture.

3.   Stir in remaining ingredients (except cocoa powder) and form small balls out of the mixture.

4.   Coat with cocoa powder, serve and enjoy!

Nutrition (Per Serving)

Calories: 265

Fat: 12g

Carbohydrates: 43g

Protein 3g

Hearty Buttery Walnuts

Serving: 4

Prep Time: 10 minutes

Cook Time: nil

Ingredients:

4 walnut halves

½ tablespoon almond butter

How To:

1. Spread butter over two walnut halves.

2. Top with other halves.

3. Serve and enjoy!

Nutrition (Per Serving)

Calories: 90

Fat: 10g

Carbohydrates: 0g

Protein: 1g

Feisty Mango and Coconut Smoothie

Serving: 2

Prep Time: 5 minutes

Ingredients:

1 teaspoon spirulina

1 cup frozen mango

1 cup unsweetened coconut milk

½ cup spinach

How To:

1.	Cut mangoes and dice them.

2.	Add mango, cup of unsweetened coconut milk, teaspoon of Spirulina and spinach to the blender.

3.	Blend on low to medium until smooth.

4.	Check the texture and serve chilled!

Nutrition (Per Serving)

Calories: 200

Fat: 10g

Carbohydrates: 14g

Protein 2g

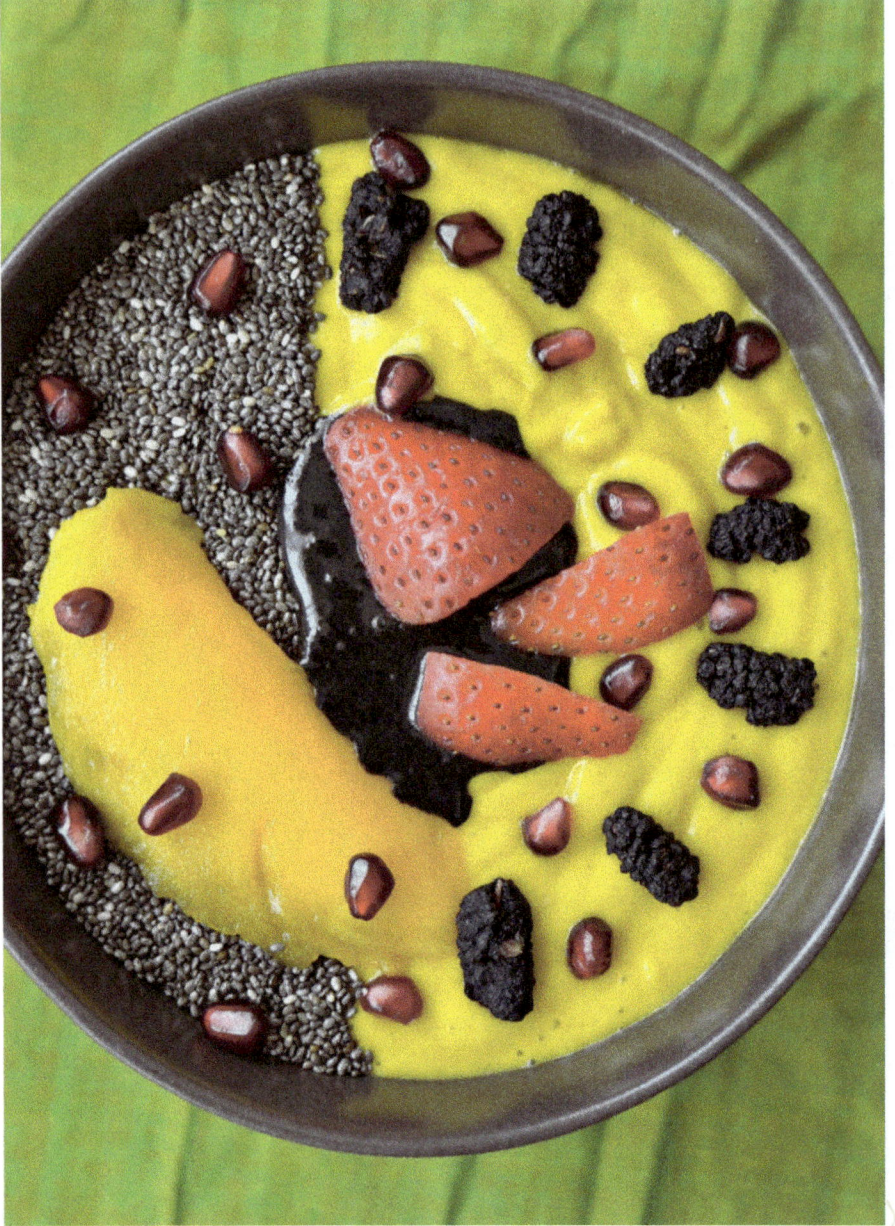

Mexican Chocolate Stand-Off

Serving: 2

Prep Time: 5 minutes

Ingredients:

2 bananas

1 tablespoon hemp seeds

1 bag frozen blueberries

½ teaspoon liquid stevia

Pure water

2 teaspoons raw chocolate

1 teaspoon raw carob powder

½ teaspoon green powder

½ teaspoon cinnamon powder

Pinch of cayenne pepper

How To:

1.   Add all the listed ingredients to your blender.

2.   Blend until smooth.

3. Add a few ice cubes and serve the smoothie.

4. Enjoy!

Nutrition (Per Serving)

Calories: 200

Fat: 10g

Carbohydrates: 14g

Protein 2g

The Awesome Cleanser

Serving: 2

Prep Time: 5 minutes

Ingredients:

2 grapefruits, juiced

2 lemons, juiced

Half cup alkaline water/filtered water

2 tablespoons olive oil

2 cucumbers, peeled

1 avocado, peeled and pitted

2 cloves fresh garlic

1-inch ginger

Pinch of Himalayan salt

Pinch of cayenne pepper

How To:

1.   Add cucumber, ginger, avocado, grapefruit and lemon to your blender.

2.   Blend until smooth.

3.   Add alkaline water, spices and oil.

4.   Stir well and drink chilled.

5.   Enjoy!

Nutrition (Per Serving)

Calories: 200

Fat: 10g

Carbohydrates: 14g

Protein 2g

Gentle Tropical Papaya Smoothie

Serving: 2

Prep Time: 5 minutes

Ingredients:

1 papaya, cut into chunks

1 cup fat free plain yogurt

½ cup pineapple chunks

½ cup crushed ice

1 teaspoon coconut extract

1 teaspoon flaxseed

How To:

1.   Add the listed ingredients to your blender and blend until smooth.

2.   Serve chilled!

Nutrition (Per Serving)

Calories: 200

Fat: 10g

Carbohydrates: 14g

Protein 2g

Kale and Apple Smoothie

Serving: 2

Prep Time: 5 minutes

Ingredients:

¾ of a kale, chopped, ribs and stem removed 1 small stalk celery, chopped ½ banana

½ cup apple juice

1 tablespoon lemon juice

How To:

1.   Add the listed ingredients to your blender and blend until smooth.

2.   Serve chilled!

Nutrition (Per Serving)

Calories: 200

Fat: 10g

Carbohydrates: 14g

Protein 2g

Mango and Lime Generous Smoothie

Serving: 2

Prep Time: 5 minutes

Ingredients:

2 tablespoons lime juice

2 cups spinach, chopped and stemmed

1 ½ cups frozen mango, cubed

1 cup green grapes

How To:

1.   Add the listed ingredients to your blender and blend until smooth

2.   Serve chilled!

Nutrition (Per Serving)

Calories: 200

Fat: 10g

Carbohydrates: 14g

Protein 2g

Juicy Summertime Veggies

Serving: 6

Prep Time: 10 minutes

Cooking Time: 3 hours 5 minutes

Ingredients:

1 cup grape tomatoes

2 cups okra

1 cup mushrooms

2 cups yellow bell peppers

1 ½ cup red onions

2 ½ cups zucchini

½ cup olive oil

½ cup balsamic vinegar

1 tablespoon fresh thyme, chopped

2 tablespoons fresh basil, chopped

How To:

1.   Slice and chop okra, onions, tomatoes, zucchini, mushrooms.

2.   Add veggies to a large container and mix.

3.   Take another dish and add oil and vinegar, mix in thyme and basil.

4.   Toss the veggies into the Slow Cooker and pour marinade.

5.   Stir well.

6.   Close lid and cook on 3 hours on HIGH, making sure to stir after every hour.

Nutrition (Per Serving)

Calories: 233

Fat: 18g

Carbohydrates: 14g

Protein: 3g

Crazy Caramelized Onion

Serving:

Prep Time: 10 minutes

Cooking Time: 9-10 hours

Ingredients:

6 onions, sliced

2 tablespoons oil

½ teaspoon salt

How To:

1.　　Add onions, oil and salt to your Slow Cooker.

2.　　Close lid and cook on LOW for 8 hours.

3.　　Open lid and keep simmering for 1-2 hours until any excess water has evaporated.

4.　　Serve and enjoy!

Nutrition (Per Serving)

Calories: 126

Fat: 15g

Carbohydrates: 15g

Protein: 2g

Kidney Beans and Cilantro

Serving: 6

Prep Time: 5 minutes

Cook Time: nil

Ingredients:

1 can (15 ounces) kidney beans, drained and rinsed ½ English cucumber, chopped

1 medium heirloom tomato, chopped

1 bunch fresh cilantro, stems removed and chopped

1 red onion, chopped

Juice of 1 large lime

3 tablespoons Dijon mustard

½ teaspoon fresh garlic paste

1 teaspoon Sumac

Salt and pepper as needed

How To:

1.   Take a medium-sized bowl and add kidney beans, chopped up veggies and cilantro.

2.   Take a small bowl and make the vinaigrette by adding lime juice, oil, fresh garlic, pepper, mustard and Sumac.

3.   Pour the vinaigrette over the salad and give it a gentle stir.

4.   Add some salt and pepper.

5.   Cover and allow to chill for half an hour.

6.   Serve!

Nutrition (Per Serving)

Calories: 74

Fat: 0.7g

Carbohydrates: 16g

Protein: 21g

Broccoli Crunchies

Serving: 4

Prep Time: 10 minutes

Cooking Time: 3 hours

Ingredients:

2 cups broccoli florets

2 ounces cream of celery soup

2 tablespoons cheddar cheese, shredded

1 small yellow onion, chopped

¼ teaspoon Worcestershire sauce

Salt and pepper as needed

½ tablespoon butter

How To:

1.   Add broccoli, cream, cheese, onion, cheddar to Slow Cooker.

2.   Stir and season with salt and pepper.

3.   Place lid and cook on LOW for 3 hours.

4.   Serve and enjoy!

Nutrition (Per Serving)

Calories: 162

Fat: 11g

Carbohydrates: 11g

Protein: 5g

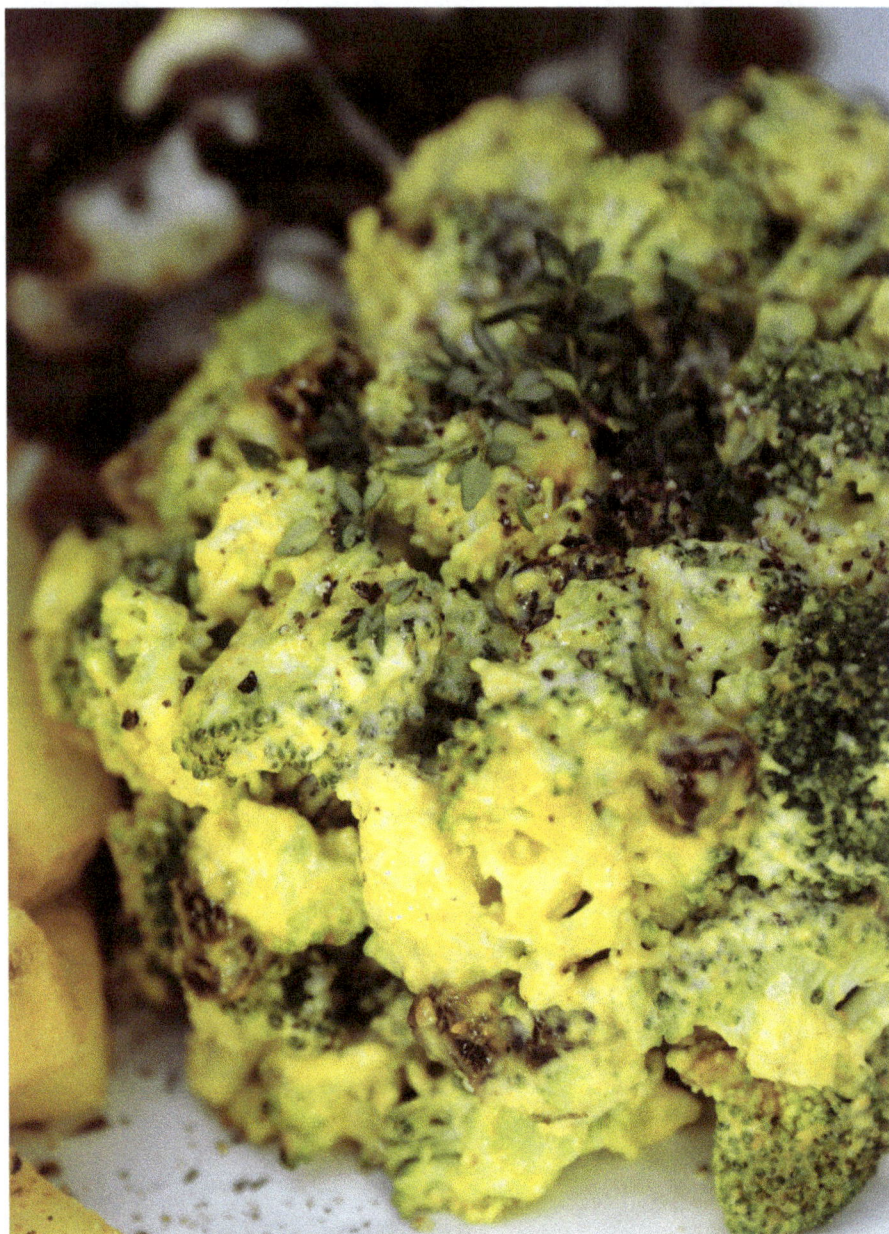

Ultimate Buffalo Cashews

Serving: 4

Prep Time: 10 minutes

Cook Time: 55 minutes

Ingredients:

2 cups raw cashews

¾ cup red hot sauce

1/3 cup avocado oil

½ teaspoon garlic powder

¼ teaspoon turmeric

How To:

1.   Take a bowl, mix the wet ingredients in a bowl and stir in seasoning.

2.   Add cashews to the bowl and mix.

3.   Soak cashews in hot sauce mix for 2-4 hours.

4.   Pre-heat your oven to 325 degrees F.

5.   Spread cashews onto baking sheet.

6. Bake for 35-55 minutes, turning after every 10-15 minutes.

7. Let them cool and serve!

Nutrition (Per Serving)

Calories: 268

Fat: 16g

Carbohydrates: 20g

Protein: 14g

A Green Bean Mixture

Serving: 2

Prep Time: 10 minutes

Cooking Time: 2 hours

Ingredients:

4 cups green beans, trimmed

2 tablespoons butter, melted

1 tablespoon date paste

Salt and pepper as needed

¼ teaspoon coconut aminos

How To:

1.   Add green beans, date paste, pepper, salt, coconut aminos to the Slow Cooker, gently stir.

2.   Toss and place lid.

3.   Cook on LOW for 2 hours.

4.   Serve and enjoy!

Nutrition (Per Serving)

Calories: 236

Fat: 6g

Carbohydrates: 10g

Protein: 6g

www.ingramcontent.com/pod-product-compliance
Lightning Source LLC
Chambersburg PA
CBHW050750030426
42336CB00012B/1753